Contents

Abstract

"Whisker Wellness: A Comprehensive Guide to Feline Dental Care" is a definitive resource for cat owners, presenting an in-depth exploration of the vital role dental health plays in the overall well-being and longevity of feline companions. This guide transcends the pursuit of minty fresh breath, focusing on proactive strategies for preventing and addressing common oral conditions, essential at-home dental care practices, the significance of professional veterinary cleanings, and approaches to combatting stained teeth.

The guide begins by highlighting the broader implications of feline dental health, beyond cosmetic concerns, emphasizing its direct link to a cat's overall quality of life. Common oral conditions, such as tooth resorption, fractured teeth, deciduous tooth challenges, and dental malocclusions, are examined with a focus on early identification and intervention.

Essential dental care practices, including the gradual introduction of toothbrushing and alternative care options, provide practical guidance for cat owners seeking to establish proactive dental care routines. The guide further underscores the pivotal role of professional veterinary cleanings, elucidating their complementarity to at-home care and their ability to detect unnoticed oral problems.

Addressing stained teeth in cats is a key focus, emphasizing the importance of regular toothbrushing and the role of professional veterinary dental care in managing severe stains. The guide concludes with a recap of key takeaways and a call to action, urging cat owners to prioritize their feline companion's dental care for a lifetime of whisker wellness.

"Whisker Wellness" serves as a comprehensive manual, empowering cat owners with the knowledge and practices needed to ensure optimal oral health, a brighter smile, and an enhanced quality of life for their cherished feline

friends.

.

Introduction

Welcome to "Whisker Wellness: A Comprehensive Guide to Feline Dental Care," a definitive resource designed to empower cat owners with the knowledge and practices necessary for ensuring the optimal dental health of their feline companions. In the world of feline care, the significance of dental well-being extends far beyond aesthetics, playing a pivotal role in a cat's overall health, longevity, and quality of life.

Chapter 1 of this guide establishes the groundwork by exploring the broader implications of feline dental health, moving beyond the pursuit of minty fresh breath to illuminate the profound impact good dental hygiene has on the well-being of our beloved cats. From identifying common oral conditions, such as tooth resorption and fractured teeth, to understanding the challenges posed by deciduous teeth and dental malocclusions, this chapter sets the stage for proactive and informed care.

Chapter 2 delves into essential dental care practices for cats, with a particular focus on the gold standard—brushing your cat's teeth. The guide provides practical advice on choosing the right tools, introducing toothbrushing gradually, and creating positive associations to make this essential practice a manageable and positive experience for both owner and feline friend.

Chapter 3 introduces alternative dental care options for cats, recognizing that every cat is unique and may require varied approaches to dental care. From dental chews and treats to sprays and interactive toys, this chapter explores diverse avenues to cater to different preferences and needs.

In Chapter 4, the guide emphasizes the necessity of professional veterinary cleanings as a crucial complement to at-home care. Understanding what occurs during a veterinary cleaning, the frequency of cleanings, and the importance of scaling, polishing, and dental radiographs provides cat owners with insights into the comprehensive nature of professional dental care.

Chapter 5 addresses the common concern of stained teeth in cats. It underscores the importance of regular toothbrushing in preventing stains and explores the role of professional veterinary dental care in managing severe stains. This chapter encapsulates the guide's commitment to a proactive approach to feline dental care.

In the concluding chapter, we recap key takeaways and issue a call to action, urging cat owners to invest time and effort into their cat's dental care. By prioritizing whisker wellness, cat owners embark on a journey toward a lifetime of optimal oral health, a brighter smile, and an enduring bond with their feline companions.

Join us as we navigate the world of feline dental care, where each chapter serves as a stepping stone towards a healthier, happier, and more vibrant life for your cherished cat.

Chapter One

The Importance of Feline Dental Health

Beyond Minty Freshness

The significance of feline dental health transcends the desire for minty fresh breath. Cats, known for their independent and stoic nature, often conceal signs of oral discomfort, making it crucial for pet owners to understand the broader implications of good dental hygiene.

Dental health in cats is directly linked to their overall well-being and longevity.

While a cat's breath might not always be as fragrant as a field of flowers, it serves as a diagnostic tool for attentive owners. Foul odors can be indicative of dental issues, ranging from plaque and tartar buildup to more severe conditions like gingivitis or periodontal disease. Addressing these concerns promptly not only ensures a more pleasant living environment but also safeguards against potential systemic health problems.

Link to Overall Well-being and Longevity

Maintaining proper feline dental health contributes significantly to a cat's overall well-being and can impact their lifespan. Dental issues, if left untreated, can lead to pain, difficulty eating, and a reduced quality of life for our feline friends. Furthermore, the correlation between oral health and systemic conditions in cats underscores the importance of proactive dental care.

Studies have shown that cats with good oral hygiene are more likely to live longer, healthier lives. This is attributed to the prevention of secondary health issues that can arise from neglected dental care. By prioritizing and practicing regular dental care, cat owners are not only preserving their feline companion's teeth and gums but also promoting a higher standard of living.

Common Dental Issues in Cats

Understanding common dental issues in cats is essential for proactive care and early intervention. The following are some prevalent oral conditions in felines:

Tooth Resorption in Cats

This condition involves the breakdown and loss of tooth structure, often causing pain and discomfort. Identifying tooth resorption early is crucial for preventing further complications.

Fractured Feline Teeth

Cats, known for their agility and curiosity, may experience fractured teeth due to accidents or chewing on hard objects. Fractured teeth can lead to pain and the risk of infection if not addressed promptly.

Challenges with Deciduous Teeth

Similar to dogs, some cats may retain their deciduous (baby) teeth, leading to misalignments and potential oral health issues. Timely identification and extraction of retained deciduous teeth are necessary for proper dental development.

Addressing Dental Malocclusions in Cats

Misalignments of the teeth and jaws, known as dental malocclusions, can affect a cat's ability to eat comfortably. Identifying and addressing malocclusions may involve orthodontic measures, extractions, or other corrective treatments.

Recognizing the importance of feline dental health sets the foundation for a proactive approach to care. In the subsequent chapters, we will delve into essential dental care practices, alternative options for at-home care, and the role of professional veterinary cleanings in ensuring your cat enjoys a lifetime of optimal oral health.

Chapter Two

Recognizing Feline Oral Conditions

Tooth Resorption in Cats

Tooth resorption is a common and often painful dental issue in cats that involves the gradual breakdown and loss of tooth structure. This condition, also known as feline odontoclastic resorptive lesions (FORL), can affect cats of all ages and breeds. Recognizing the signs of tooth resorption is crucial for early intervention and preventing unnecessary discomfort for your feline companion.

Signs of tooth resorption may include changes in eating habits, increased salivation, pawing at the mouth, and reluctance to allow mouth examination. Routine dental check-ups are essential for early detection, and dental X-rays are often necessary to assess the extent of resorption below the gumline. Veterinary intervention, including tooth extraction if needed, can alleviate pain and improve your cat's oral health.

Fractured Feline Teeth

Cats are curious and agile creatures, but their adventurous spirit can sometimes lead to fractured teeth. Fractures can range from minor chips to more severe breaks that expose the sensitive pulp chamber. Cats may exhibit signs of dental pain, such as reluctance to eat, drooling, or changes in behavior.

Early identification of fractured teeth is vital for preventing complications such as infections. A thorough dental examination by a veterinarian, possibly including dental X-rays, can help assess the extent of the fracture and guide appropriate treatment. Treatment options may include bonding, crowns, or in severe cases, extraction to alleviate pain and prevent further issues.

Challenges with Deciduous Teeth

Just like in dogs, some cats may experience challenges with deciduous (baby) teeth not falling out naturally. Retained deciduous teeth can lead to misalignments and impact the proper development of permanent teeth. Timely identification and extraction of retained deciduous teeth are crucial for preventing issues such as malocclusions and maintaining a healthy dentition.

Observing your kitten's dental development and seeking guidance from your veterinarian can aid in identifying and addressing challenges with deciduous teeth. Early intervention ensures the successful eruption of permanent teeth and sets the stage for a lifetime of good oral health.

Addressing Dental Malocclusions in Cats

Dental malocclusions, or misalignments of the teeth and jaws, can affect a cat's ability to eat comfortably. While some malocclusions are congenital, others may develop over time. Different cat breeds may be predisposed to specific malocclusions, emphasizing the need for breed-specific dental care.

Identifying dental malocclusions involves a comprehensive dental examination, and dental X-rays may be necessary to assess the alignment of the teeth below the gumline. Treatment options depend on the nature and severity of the malocclusion and may include orthodontic devices, extractions, or other corrective measures.

By recognizing these common oral conditions in cats and being proactive in seeking veterinary care, cat owners can ensure their feline companions maintain optimal oral health. In the following chapters, we will delve into essential dental care practices that can be implemented at home to prevent these conditions and promote a lifetime of whisker wellness for your cat.

Chapter Three

Essential Dental Care Practices for Cats

Brushing Your Cat's Teeth

Brushing your cat's teeth is a cornerstone of feline dental care, helping to prevent plaque buildup, bad breath, and dental issues. While it may seem challenging given a cat's independent nature, introducing toothbrushing gradually and using positive reinforcement can make it a manageable and positive experience.

Choosing the Right Tools

Select a cat-specific toothbrush with soft bristles and feline-friendly toothpaste. Cat toothpaste comes in flavors that appeal to cats, such as poultry or seafood, making the experience more enjoyable.

Gradual Introduction to Toothbrushing

Start by gently touching your cat's lips and then progress to rubbing their gums with your finger. Introduce the toothbrush gradually, allowing your cat to get used to the sensation. Be patient and use positive reinforcement, such as treats or praise, to create a positive association.

Frequency of Toothbrushing

Ideally, aim to brush your cat's teeth a few times per week. Consistency is key to maintaining good oral hygiene and preventing the buildup of plaque and tartar.

Alternative Dental Care Options for Cats

If traditional toothbrushing proves challenging, alternative dental care options offer effective ways to promote oral health:

Dental Chews and Treats

Specially formulated dental chews or treats can provide a tasty and enjoyable way for cats to maintain their oral health. These treats often have a texture that helps reduce plaque and tartar.

Dental Sprays

Dental sprays offer a convenient option for freshening your cat's breath and providing additional oral care between brushings. Choose sprays with cat-friendly flavors and antibacterial properties.

Interactive Toys for Dental Health

Toys that encourage chewing or contain dental ridges can contribute to oral health by reducing plaque and promoting healthy gums. Interactive toys can also provide mental stimulation for your cat.

Incorporating these alternative options into your cat's routine can make dental care more manageable and enjoyable for both you and your feline friend.

In the next section, we will explore the importance of professional veterinary cleanings as a complementary measure to at-home dental care, ensuring a comprehensive approach to your cat's oral health.

Chapter Four

Professional Dental Cleanings for Cats

The Necessity of Veterinary Cleanings

While at-home dental care practices are essential, professional cleanings by a veterinarian play a crucial role in ensuring comprehensive feline dental health. Here's why regular veterinary cleanings are indispensable:

Complementing At-Home Care

Professional dental cleanings serve as a complement to your at-home dental care efforts.

Despite diligent brushing and alternative care, certain areas of a cat's mouth may be challenging to reach or clean thoroughly. Veterinary cleanings ensure a thorough removal of plaque and tartar, particularly in areas that are difficult to access during routine home care.

Detecting Unnoticed Oral Problems

Veterinarians are trained to identify and address oral problems that may go unnoticed by pet owners. During a professional cleaning, the veterinarian can identify issues such as early signs of periodontal disease, infections, or abnormalities that may require further investigation or treatment.

Scaling, Polishing, and Radiographs

Professional dental cleanings involve a comprehensive process that goes beyond what can be achieved at home. This includes scaling to remove tartar and plaque both above and below the gumline, polishing to smooth tooth surfaces and discourage plaque buildup, and the use of dental radiographs to assess the health of the teeth and supporting structures.

Frequency of Veterinary Cleanings

The frequency of professional dental cleanings may vary based on factors such as a cat's age, breed, and overall dental health. In general, annual veterinary cleanings are recommended, but certain breeds or cats with specific oral health concerns may require more frequent cleanings.

What to Expect During a Veterinary Cleaning

Understanding what occurs during a veterinary cleaning can help alleviate concerns and emphasize the importance of this aspect of feline dental care:

General Anesthesia for Stress-Free Experience

To ensure a stress-free and safe experience, your cat will be placed under general anesthesia during the veterinary cleaning. This not only allows for a more thorough examination and cleaning but also ensures your cat remains calm and comfortable throughout the procedure.

Thorough Cleaning Below the Gumline

The veterinarian will meticulously clean your cat's teeth, paying special attention to the areas below the gumline where tartar and plaque can accumulate. This is a critical step in preventing and addressing periodontal disease, a common and often painful condition in cats.

Comprehensive Oral Examination

In addition to cleaning, the veterinarian will conduct a comprehensive oral examination. This may involve evaluating the gums, teeth, tongue, and other oral structures. Any abnormalities or issues discovered during this examination will be addressed accordingly.

Dental Radiographs and Additional Treatments

Dental radiographs (X-rays) may be taken to assess the health of the tooth roots and surrounding structures. If any dental issues are identified, such as cavities, fractures, or abscesses, appropriate treatments, such as fillings or extractions, will be performed.

Regular veterinary cleanings, combined with consistent at-home dental care practices, contribute significantly to maintaining your cat's oral health and preventing serious dental problems.

In the next section, we will explore strategies for preventing and addressing stained teeth in cats, emphasizing the importance of regular toothbrushing and professional veterinary dental care.

Chapter Five

Addressing Stained Teeth in Cats

Importance of Regular Toothbrushing

Preventing stained teeth in cats begins with regular toothbrushing. Stains can result from factors such as diet, age, and certain medications. Regular toothbrushing helps remove plaque and surface stains, promoting a cleaner and brighter smile for your feline companion.

Daily Dental Care Routine

Incorporate toothbrushing into your cat's daily routine. Use a cat-specific toothbrush and toothpaste, gradually introducing these tools to create a positive association. Regular brushing not only aids in stain prevention but also contributes to overall oral health.

Surface Stain Removal

The mechanical action of toothbrushing helps remove superficial discoloration. By staying consistent with toothbrushing, you minimize the accumulation of stains caused by food and bacteria, maintaining a healthier appearance for your cat's teeth.

Maintaining Fresh Breath

In addition to stain prevention, regular toothbrushing helps combat bad breath by reducing the bacteria responsible for oral odors.

A cat with a clean and healthy mouth is likely to have fresher breath, enhancing the overall bond between pet and owner.

Positive Reinforcement

Make toothbrushing a positive experience for your cat by offering treats or affection as a reward. This positive reinforcement creates a cooperative atmosphere, making future toothbrushing sessions more manageable.

Professional Veterinary Dental Care

If your cat's teeth are severely stained or if you encounter challenges in maintaining their oral health, seeking professional veterinary dental care is essential.

Scaling Away Tartar and Polishing

A veterinary dentist can perform a professional dental cleaning to address stubborn tartar and stains. This involves scaling to remove accumulated plaque and tartar and polishing to restore a smoother and cleaner tooth surface.

Resuming Toothbrushing Post-Professional Cleaning

While professional veterinary dental care can significantly improve the appearance of stained teeth, it's crucial to resume regular toothbrushing immediately afterward. Consistent at-home dental care is essential for maintaining the benefits of the professional cleaning and preventing future stains and oral health issues.

In summary, addressing stained teeth in cats requires a proactive approach that combines regular toothbrushing with professional veterinary dental care when needed. By prioritizing your cat's oral health, you not only enhance their appearance but also contribute to their overall well-being and longevity.

The journey to a vibrant and healthy smile for your feline friend involves consistent dental care practices, both at home and with the guidance of your veterinarian. By implementing the strategies outlined in this guide, you are taking significant steps towards ensuring your cat enjoys a lifetime of optimal oral health and a sparkling smile.

In the final section, we'll recap the key takeaways and reinforce the importance of investing time and effort into your cat's dental care.

Conclusion

Congratulations on reaching the end of "Whisker Wellness: A Comprehensive Guide to Feline Dental Care." Throughout this guide, we've delved into the significance of feline dental health, common oral conditions in cats, essential dental care practices, the importance of professional veterinary cleanings, and strategies for addressing stained teeth.

Key Takeaways

Beyond Minty Freshness

- Feline dental health is crucial for overall well-being and longevity.

- Recognizing the broader implications of good dental hygiene, beyond fresh breath, is essential for proactive care.

Common Oral Conditions

- Tooth resorption, fractured teeth, challenges with deciduous teeth, and dental malocclusions are common issues requiring early identification and intervention.

Essential Dental Care Practices

- Regular toothbrushing is a cornerstone for preventing stains, plaque, and maintaining overall oral health.

- Alternative options like dental chews, sprays, and interactive toys provide additional avenues for at-home care.

Professional Veterinary Cleanings

- Regular cleanings by a veterinarian complement at-home care, ensuring thorough removal of plaque and tartar.

- Professional dental care detects and addresses unnoticed oral problems, contributing to long-term feline health.

Addressing Stained Teeth

- Regular toothbrushing is instrumental in preventing and managing stained teeth.

- Professional veterinary dental care helps address severe stains, with a need for consistent at-home care post-cleaning.

Conclusion and Call to Action

By prioritizing your cat's dental care, you are investing in their immediate comfort and long-term health. Regular toothbrushing, alternative care options, and professional veterinary cleanings collectively form a comprehensive approach to feline dental wellness.

Remember

- Dental care should start early, ideally in kittenhood.
- Different cat breeds may have specific dental needs.

- Consult with your veterinarian for personalized dental care advice tailored to your feline companion.

Investing time and effort into your cat's dental care is a gift that keeps on giving—a lifetime of optimal oral health and a radiant smile. May your cat's whiskers always shine bright!

Thank you for embarking on this journey towards whisker wellness with us.